Activities for the Family Caregiver

DEMENTIA

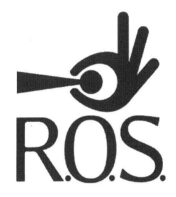

R.O.S.

HOW TO ENGAGE
HOW TO LIVE

Scott Silknitter
Robert D. Brennan, RN, NHA, MS, CDP
Dawn Worsley, ADC/MC/EDU, CDP

Disclaimer

This book is for informational purposes only and is not intended as medical advice, diagnosis, or treatment. Always seek advice from a qualified physician about medical concerns, and do not disregard medical advice because of something you may read within this book. This book does not replace the need for diagnostic evaluation, ongoing physician care, and professional assessment of treatments. Every effort has been made to make this book as complete and helpful as possible. It is important, however, for this book to be used as a resource and idea-generating guide and not as an ultimate source for plan of care.

ISBN 978-1-943285-96-9

Published by
R.O.S. Therapy Systems, L.L.C.
Greensboro, NC
888-352-9788
www.ROSTherapySystems.com

Activities for the Family Caregiver – Dementia

This book is a general guide to Activities for the Family Caregiver of someone with dementia. It is based on the principles and approaches used in the training of professional staff in long-term care settings. It is part of the R.O.S. Activities 101 and 201 Programs that will help you engage your senior loved one in meaningful activities.

With the assistance of Robert D. Brennan, RN, NHA, MS, CDP, and Dawn Worsley, ADC/MC/EDU, CDP, who have been working in long-term care for a combined 60 years, we have written this book for you with the hope of providing helpful information on caregiving, activities of daily living and taking care of yourself.

We hope you find the educational information and activity suggestions useful. We encourage you to have other family members and caregivers of your loved one read this book in order to be consistent with approaches, verbal cues, physical assistance and modifications that produce positive results.

From our family of caregivers to yours, please remember that you are not alone, and to never give up.

Scott Silknitter

**Family Members and Caregivers
that have read this book:**

_____

_____

_____

_____

_____

_____

_____

_____

_____

_____

Table of Contents

Chapter 1

Dementia Overview and Symptoms

Dementia is not actually a disease. It is a collection of symptoms that can be caused by various diseases or injury. Dementia involves damage of nerve cells in the brain. This damage may occur in different areas of the brain causing dementia which may affect people differently.

In the most simplistic explanation, dementia causes problems with memory, communication and thinking.

Back in the day, dementia might have been associated with the word "senile." Someone experiencing memory loss while trying to locate their keys, or remember someone's name, may be said to be "having a senior moment."

Regardless of how it is described, dementia is a struggle for everyone involved: your loved one, you as the caregiver, family and friends.

Your loved one did not choose to have dementia. You did not choose to become a caregiver. But they have both happened and you must be prepared to work with and adapt to the changes occurring in your loved one.

Dementia can be looked at in one of two ways: reversible and irreversible.

Some dementias can be caused by things like reaction to a medication, vitamin deficiency, depression, or an infection that can be reversed through treatment.

Dementias that are not reversible and get worse over time can be caused by a variety of issues and diseases. Dementias can be classified in several ways and are often grouped by what they have in common, such as what part of the brain is affected, or whether they worsen over time (progressive dementias).

Some of the most common symptoms of dementia that your loved one may experience and examples are:

Memory Loss

- Forgetting where their eyeglasses are
- Forgetting appointments
- Forgetting they have retired
- Forgetting they have kids
- Forgetting they are an adult that does not live with their parents anymore

Difficulty with Communication

- Cannot find the right words to tell you things such as having to go to the bathroom or what they would like to eat

Poor Judgment

- Making choices that put their safety at risk such as being out in the cold without a jacket

- Inability to determine the important from the unimportant

- Misjudging the intentions of others

- Giving away large sums of money

- Neglecting personal care and safety

Difficulty Planning and Organizing

- Making dinner or lunch
    - ° Deciding what to eat
    - ° Finding ingredients in the cabinet or refrigerator
    - ° Making a list of ingredients needed at the grocery store

Difficulty with Orientation

- Getting lost easily

- Inability to find way back home

Coordination and Motor Function Issues

- Losing their balance

- Trouble with walking, stepping or running (gait)

- Difficulty picking items up from floor
- Difficulty folding clothes

Personality Changes

- May withdraw from family conversations
- May become easily frustrated
- May become argumentative and defensive as a way not to let the family know how much the dementia has affected their abilities
- May become more sarcastic making everything into a joke

Inability to Reason

- Not understanding why they have to get washed up/showered
- Not understanding why they can't go outside even though it is cold and raining
- Not wanting to take their medicine because they think they have already taken it

Inappropriate Behavior

- Taking things that do not belong to them

- Inappropriate sexual comments

- Demanding and making unreasonable requests

- Not compliant with "normal" social conduct, such as talking loudly in church

- Saying things that we usually only think but would never say to someone

Paranoia, Agitation, Hallucinations

- Thinking that others are talking about them

- Not wanting to take medicine or eat, claiming someone has poisoned it

- Frustrations quickly turning to aggressive verbal or physical behavior

- Misinterpreting sounds in the house even after explanation of what it was

Common Diseases
That Cause Dementia

There are many types of dementia-causing diseases or issues, but the most common forms are:

Alzheimer's Disease

The most common cause of dementia, Alzheimer's disease, usually progresses over an eight to ten-year period. Your loved one's cognitive ability slowly declines affecting parts of their brain that affect:

- Memory

    The initial symptom of Alzheimer's disease is memory loss. Your loved one may remember what the buttercream frosting on your wedding cake tasted like on your wedding day, but may not be able to remember what they ate for breakfast.

- Language

  Communication can be a significant challenge with dementia. For your loved one, it may be something as simple as not being able to find the "right" word to describe something or not finding the words to use at all. For example, using the word "horses" when describing cars on the road.

- Judgment

  Your loved one's judgment may be affected in several ways with dementia, including making choices that put their safety at risk either physically or financially. This may be something as simple as trying to grab a hot pan that has been on the stove all day or trying to get out of a moving car.

- Spatial Abilities

  Spatial abilities are those that allow a person to think or visualize items three dimensionally and solve problems. For example, they are trying to walk in the house from a carpeted area to a tile area and they think they have to step down or step up. Another example is that a black welcome mat could appear as a hole and your loved one may try to step over it or walk around it.

Vascular Dementia

Vascular dementia is the second most common type of dementia. It is caused by damage to the brain due to blocked or reduced blood flow in blood vessels leading to the brain. This may be a result of a stroke, heart valve condition or another blood vessel condition.

Lewy Body Dementia

Symptoms of Lewy body dementia (LBD) are similar to those of Alzheimer's disease. Some unique features of LBD include fluctuations between confusion and clear thinking, visual hallucinations, and tremor and rigidity.

Frontal Lobe / Frontotemporal Dementia / Pick's Disease

This dementia is a group of disorders characterized by the breakdown of nerve cells in the frontal and temporal lobes of the brain, which are areas generally associated with personality, behavior and language. At one time, the dementia symptoms associated with frontotemporal dementia were also known as Pick's disease. Some still use the term Pick's disease today.

Unique symptoms of frontal lobe / fronto-temporal dementia include inappropriate behaviors, language problems, and difficulty with thinking, concentration and movement.

The behavior and language problem is why some call this "The Terse and Curse" dementia. In other words, not many words are said, but what comes out of your loved one's mouth may be things you may not be accustomed to hearing such as swearing.

Other Causes of Dementia

Huntington's Disease

Signs and symptoms usually appear during your 30s or 40s. People may experience personality changes, such as irritability or anxiety.

The condition causes a severe decline in thinking (cognitive) skills over time. Huntington's disease also causes weakness and difficulty with walking and movement.

Traumatic Brain Injury

This condition is caused by head trauma. It can be experienced by those with repeated blows to the head such as football players or boxers. It can also be experienced by those with a single massive blow to the head such as members of the military or someone who falls and hits their head on the ground.

Depending on the part of the brain that is injured, this can cause dementia symptoms such as memory loss, uncoordinated movement and impaired speech, as well as slow movement, tremors and rigidity. Symptoms may not appear until many years after the injury.

Creutzfeldt-Jakob Disease

This rare brain disorder usually occurs in people without risk factors. It may be due to an abnormal form of a protein. Creutzfeldt-Jakob disease sometimes may be inherited or caused by exposure to diseased brain or nervous system tissue.

Signs and symptoms of this fatal condition usually appear around age 60 and include problems with coordination, memory, thinking and vision. Symptoms worsen over time and may include the inability to move, talk and possibly blindness.

Parkinson's Disease

Many people with Parkinson's disease eventually develop dementia symptoms. For more information on Parkinson's disease, please read the R.O.S. book *Activities 101 for the Family Caregiver – Parkinson's Disease.*

No matter the cause, there are several general symptoms that your loved one may experience. As the primary caregiver, you must be as prepared and flexible as possible to handle them. On any given day, you may not know what kind of day you will have until your loved one is awake and the day has begun. If you notice that something is different and that they are starting on the path to a "bad day," look for any reason, no matter how small, that could be the trigger.

Now that we have reviewed what some of the symptoms of your loved one's dementia might be, let's talk about the "how to's," preparation and execution of activities for your loved one.

Chapter 2

Activities, Their Benefits and the Family

"Activities" and "Activities of Daily Living" (ADLs) are critical aspects to caring for a loved one at home. Both types, leisure and daily living, require knowledge of your loved one's habits, preferences, abilities and routines. This knowledge will enhance the ability of all caregivers to communicate and execute a planned activity with your loved one. Life happens and things can happen spontaneously, but all activities should be planned to offer the best possible outcome to enhance your loved one's sense of well-being and to promote or enhance their physical, cognitive and emotional health. In this book, we will focus on leisure activities and the activities of daily living with common sense suggestions and tips on the "how to's" of getting your loved one engaged, dressed or fed.

In the institutional setting of today, Leisure Activities are required by law if a nursing home accepts government funding. In these situations, Activities are to be provided to every resident on a daily basis based on an individual's preferences. Activities has grown into a profession where Certified Activity Professionals and their staff plan and execute leisure activity programs for residents and seniors in their care. It is NOT just bingo.

In addition, staff members are required to undergo annual training on the basics of Activities of Daily Living in order to provide better care for the residents they work with.

This book was made for the millions of families and informal caregivers who care for their loved ones with some form of dementia at home. Recognizing the growth in the numbers of those aging in place due to financial need or desire to just be at home, the R.O.S. Activities 101/201 Programs and this book are based on the principles and

approaches used by the professionals
in skilled settings. This was done for
two reasons.

1. Provide family caregivers the knowledge
   and tools to allow them to engage their
   loved one so that both can enjoy the
   benefits of activities.

2. Offer a starting point that will provide
   continuity of approach, care,
   communication and information-gathering
   to minimize changes and acclimation time
   if your loved one does have to move from
   home to an institutional setting.

If you choose to use the services of a home
care agency while caring for your loved one at
home, please ask if they have a Home Care
Certified professional on staff and make sure
that the caregiver you choose has received
basic training on Leisure Activities and
Activities of Daily Living. This will assist with
continuity of approach, communication and
planning that will benefit both you and your
loved one.

Our goal is to help you deliver meaningful programs of interest to your loved one that focus on physical, social, spiritual, cognitive and recreational activities. Everyone involved in the care for your loved one should be "on the same page" to minimize changes and challenges that your loved one will face.

Not all family members may understand or accept your loved one's dementia or disease. Your loved one may look the same on the outside and might be having a "good day" when someone comes to visit. Family members who visit occasionally may not understand or see all of the symptoms that primary caregivers see daily. They may underestimate or minimize the responsibilities or stress. This can create conflict. If it helps to avoid a conflict or stress, please have the family members read this book prior to a visit so they can begin to understand the monumental task that you face as a caregiver. Use visits and interactions as teaching moments and to let the visitors know that they will not "catch it" just from being around your loved one.

It can take a while to learn new roles and responsibilities. It is critical, however, to have as many family members and friends involved in your loved one's life as possible. This is not just to show your loved one they are cared for and loved, but also to give you, the primary family caregiver, the occasional and much-needed break.

The importance of understanding your family dynamics and the role each individual plays in the family will lead to better understanding and comprehension for the future. As the dementia progresses, roles will evolve, and everyone needs to understand that.

Whether they come for an occasional visit or visit regularly every week, each family member can play an important role in your loved one's life. Family members can help with caregiving, preparing the home to ensure safety and quality of life, and successfully engaging with the loved one you care for.

The Benefits of Activities
with a Standard Approach

Caregiver Benefits

Planned and well-executed activities result in less stress for the caregiver as well as less stress for your loved one. Whether it is playing a game or bathing, a standard approach where as many details are planned as possible, can make a significant, positive difference for everyone.

Social Benefits of Activities

Activities offer the opportunity for increased social interaction between family members, friends, caregivers and the one being cared for. Activities create positive experiences and memories for everyone.

Behavioral Benefits of Activities

Well-planned and well-executed activities of any type can reduce challenging behaviors that sometimes arise when caring for someone with dementia.

Self-Esteem Benefits of Activities

Leisure activities offered at the right skill level provide your loved one with an opportunity for success. This is also true with Activities of Daily Living such as dressing. Success during activities improves how your loved one feels about themselves.

Sleep Benefits of Activities

As part of a daily routine, activities can improve sleeping at night. If a loved one is inactive all day, it is likely they will nap periodically. Napping can interrupt good sleep patterns at night.

Being a primary caregiver is a 24/7 job. Without help, you are always on call and run the risk of becoming physically and mentally exhausted.

When you do bring in help, make sure all of your loved one's caregivers (full-time, part-time, family and friends) use the same approach for activities and interaction that you do. With a common approach, there are significantly less opportunities to disrupt routines and make unsettling changes that affect you and your loved one long after the help has left.

A common approach is key. Demand it!

The Four Pillars of Activities

The R.O.S. Activities 101/201 Programs focus on the Four Pillars of Activities. These are areas that all caregivers for your loved one should be familiar with to provide continuity of care and give your loved one the greatest opportunity for success to engage and improve the quality of life for everyone.

1st Pillar of Activities:
Know your Loved One – Information Gathering and Assessment

Have a Personal History Form completed. Know them – who they are, who they were, and what their functional abilities are today. Make sure all caregivers know this as well.

2nd Pillar of Activities:
Communicating and Motivating for Success

Communication is key. Each caregiver must know how to effectively communicate with your loved one and be consistent with techniques.

3rd Pillar of Activities:
Customary Routines and Preferences

As best as possible, maintain a routine and daily plan based on your loved one's needs and preferences.

4th Pillar of Activities:
Planning and Executing Activities

Based on all of the information you have gathered about your loved one, you have the opportunity to offer engaging activities that are appropriate and meet your loved one's personal preferences.

Chapter 3

Home Preparation

Whether you live in a house, an apartment, or an independent living facility, you and your loved one need to feel comfortable, capable and safe. This is a key foundational piece of preparing to have your loved one engage in an activity. The following are general tips that caregivers and family members can use to prepare the home as your loved one's dementia progresses.

General Organization and Environment

When organizing your loved one's environment, be sure to do it <u>with</u> them. What works for you, may not work for your loved one.

- Assign everything to a place in the home. Always put items back in their place after using them in order to avoid clutter.

- Remove objects left on the floor, such as shoes, bags and boxes. They should be placed in their designated areas of the home. If left out, they can be a tripping hazard.

- Use extension cords sparingly and always secure them out of the places where people walk. Bundle all the cords and secure them to the wall instead of the floor.

- Organize like objects in the same area whenever possible so that they are easily located.

- Remove and avoid clutter on desks, tables and countertops, and in cabinets and closets. This makes it easier to locate and reach specific items.

- Avoid the use of throw rugs. They can be a tripping hazard when moving from room to room for an activity. If you must use them, opt for slide resistant rugs that can be taped or tacked down.

- Install handrails where possible for easier independent movement from one room to the next.

- Leave doors fully opened or closed. Make sure the doors open easily and smoothly and that doorknobs are securely fastened to the door.

- Identify and address flooring issues. Check every floor, walkway, threshold and entry. Remove or fix loose floorboards, uneven tiles, loose nails, or carpeting that has bunched up over time.

Furniture

- Make sure there is enough room to move around. If your loved one uses a wheelchair, and if possible, place furniture pieces 5½ feet from each other so your loved one can move comfortably around the room.

- Use chairs with straight backs, armrests and firm seats. Where possible, add firm cushions to existing pieces to add height. This will make it easier for your loved one to sit down and get up.

Lighting

Depending on your loved one's eye condition, dementia symptoms or individual preference, the need for additional or less lighting could be key in their safety and ability to perform tasks independently.

- Fluorescent lighting can contribute to an increase in glare. Try different types of bulbs to see which is most comfortable for your loved one.

- Keep all rooms evenly lit and lighting level consistent throughout the house so shadows and dangerous bright spots are eliminated.

- Make sure light switches, pull cords and lamps are easily accessible for your loved one in case they are in a wheelchair.

- If possible, purchase touch lamps or those that can be turned on or off by sound.

- Depending on the individual, additional task lighting may be necessary in certain areas of the home.

Glare

Glare can be caused by sunlight or light from a lamp. Glare can make it difficult for an individual with low vision to see when the glare hits shiny surfaces, including glossy paint on walls. Sunglasses can be beneficial both indoors and outside for someone who is light sensitive.

- Enable sunlight to fill the room with light without producing glare. Adjust sunlight coming from windows by using mini blinds and altering their position throughout the day. If mini blinds are not available, use sheer curtains.

- Be aware when placing mirrors in a room. Mirrors placed across from larger windows can significantly increase the amount of light in a room, but they can also be the source of a significant amount of glare.

- Cover bare lightbulbs of all types with shades.

- Position chairs and tables so that when your loved one is sitting on a chair or at a table, they are not having to look directly at the light coming from the window.

- Cover or remove shiny/reflective surfaces such as floors and tabletops.

Color Contrasts

Using contrast is a key strategy if your loved one has a visual impairment. The more contrast, the easier it is to find and use objects or activity items around the house.

- Put light-colored objects against a dark background.

- Avoid upholstery with patterns for seated activities. Stripes, plaids and checks can be visually confusing.

- Opt for solid-colored tables and countertops in a neutral tone. Countertops with busy patterns can make it difficult to locate items and can be more difficult to keep clean.

- In a room with mostly dark tones, place light-colored pillows or chairs in strategic places to help your loved one find things and get around easily.

Chapter 4

Information Gathering and Assessment

It is important, before you begin providing personal care, that you first recognize various personal attributes and abilities of your loved one and yourself. The more you know about your loved one's lifestyle, likes and dislikes, the easier providing for their personal and leisure needs will be.

Dementia may not affect your loved one's personality, but does affect their ability to interpret and deal with their surroundings as they did in the past.

It is important to concentrate on what your loved one **CAN DO**, not on what they **CAN NOT DO**. So, the more you know about your loved one, the more effective you can be as a caregiver. Caregiving routines should be kept structured and regular.

Dementia is a physical illness, not a mental illness. However, individuals may suffer from both.

Knowing your loved one is the First Pillar of Activities. Knowing their individual needs, interests, functional abilities and capacities will assist you in knowing how to communicate with them and plan or engage in activities with them.

You and your loved one may have been very private people. Having dementia will change that. Gathering information and sharing with other caregivers is critical as your loved one's past pleasures, likes and activities will become cornerstones of the communication process for everyone.

If there is something that you might consider embarrassing or private and choose not to share what happened years ago, please note that one way or another, it will come out.

Whatever it was that you think is difficult to share, caregivers and family members that offer assistance are not there to judge you or your loved one on something that happened years or even decades ago. They are there to help you in your moment of need today. Knowing your loved one is vital to the communication process and allows all caregivers the opportunity to turn a "bad" day into a "good" day through proper communication techniques.

As the primary caregiver, you may already know most of the answers, but this is a good and necessary exercise for you, other family members, and other caregivers to execute. We suggest everyone fill out the R.O.S. Personal History Form which comes later in this section, but as a starting point, you, the primary caregiver, are most likely able to provide the following basic information:

Basic Information

Name, preferred name to be called, age and date of birth

Background Information

Place of birth, cultural/ethnic background, marital status, children (how many, and their names), religion/church, military service/employment, education level and primary language spoken

Medical and Dietary/Nutritional Information

Any formal diagnosis, allergies and food regimen/diets

Habits

Drinking/alcohol, smoking, exercise and other things that are a daily habit

Physical Status

Abilities/limitations, visual aids, hearing deficits, speech, communication, hand dominance and mobility/gait

Mental Status

Alertness, cognitive abilities/limitations, orientation to family, time, place, person, routine, etc.

Social Status

One-on-one interaction, being visited, communicating with others through written word or phone calls, other means

Emotional Status

Level of contentment, outgoing/withdrawn, extroverted/introverted, dependent/independent

Leisure Status

Past, present and possible future interests

Vision Status

Any impairment they may have

Informal Assessments

Informal assessments are done through interviews, observation and information gathered through other means. These will allow you and others to "fill in the blanks" of the R.O.S. Personal History Form.

Interviews

Interviews are conducted with your loved one, or with family members, friends or significant others.

Observation

An observation is what you and others have seen or heard concerning your loved one, e.g., how they interact with others, their behavior, their responses to questions or statements made by others. This includes body language and expressions. You have probably seen these interactions a thousand times and made a mental note whenever something stuck out. Now, you must write them down for your future use and for others.

Activity Preferences

Activities are a way for individuals to establish meaning in their lives. The <u>need</u> for enjoyable activities does not change with age or growing health needs. The only thing that changes is the level of assistance individuals may need in order to engage in those pursuits.

A lack of opportunity to engage in meaningful and enjoyable activities can result in boredom, depression and behavioral disturbances.

Individuals vary in the activities they prefer, reflecting unique personalities, past interests, perceived environmental constraints, religious and cultural background, and changing physical and mental abilities. We as family caregivers have a great opportunity to empower a loved one to see that they possess many great talents and abilities. By modifying or adapting the activity to allow them to engage at an independent level, you are restoring their self-esteem and self-worth.

Your ability to identify past preferences is vital to the planning and execution of an activity, which we will cover in this book. Details matter. Let's look at someone who enjoys playing cards.

During their assessments, four people might all say they like "playing cards," yet they might not actually have the same activity in mind.

- Person 1 – Enjoys playing euchre or gin every Wednesday night with friends and family.

- Person 2 – Enjoys Friday poker night with friends.

- Person 3 – Enjoys playing solitaire with cards or on a computer.

- Person 4 – Enjoys performing card tricks.

As you can see from these examples, details matter. Gather as much information as you can for yourself and all caregivers who may help with your loved one.

The following R.O.S. Personal History Form is a starting point to gather as much information as possible.

Personal History Form

This is _____ *'s Personal History*

Name: _____

Maiden Name: _____

Date of Birth: _____

Preferred Name: _____

Name and relationship of people completing this history:

_____

_____

_____

What age do you think the person thinks they are?

_____

Do they ask for their spouse but do not recognize them?

_____

Do they look for their children but do not recognize them?

_____

Do they look for their mom? _____

Do they perceive themselves as younger? Please describe.

_____

_____

Describe the "home" they remember. _____

_____

_____

_____

Describe the person's personality prior to the onset of

dementia. _____

_____

_____

What makes the person feel valued? Talents, occupation,

accomplishments, family, etc. _____

_____

_____

What are some favorite items they must always have in

sight or close by? _____

_____

_____

What is their exact morning daily routine? _____

_____

_____

_____

_____

What is their exact evening routine?

_____

_____

_____

_____

What type of clothing do they prefer? Do they like to choose their own clothes for the day or do they prefer to have their clothes laid out for them?

_____

_____

_____

_____

What is their favorite beverage?

_____

What is their favorite food?

_____

What will get them motivated? (Church, friends coming over, going out, etc.)

_____

_____

_____

_____

List significant interests in their life, such as hobbies, recreational activities, job related skills/experiences, military experience, etc.

    - Age 8 to 20:

_____

_____

_____

    - Age 20 to 40:

_____

_____

_____

What is their religious background? (Affiliation, prayer time, symbols, traditions, church/synagogue name, etc. Did they lead any services or sing in the choir?)

_____

_____

_____

What type of music do they enjoy listening to, playing, or singing? Do they have any musical talents?

_____

_____

_____

What is their favorite TV program? Movie?

_____

_____

_____

Did they enjoy reading? Which authors, topics, or genres
do they prefer? Would they listen to audiobooks or
books on tape?

_____

_____

_____

_____

Can they tell the difference between someone on TV and
a real person?

_____

_____

Marital status - If married more than once, provide
specifics. Include names of spouses, dates of marriage and
other relevant information.

_____

_____

_____

_____

_____

List distinct characteristics about their spouse(s), such as occupations, personality traits, or daily routine.

_____

_____

_____

_____

_____

Do they have children? Be sure to include children both living and deceased. Include names, birth dates and any other relevant information.

_____

_____

_____

_____

_____

Who do they ask for the most? What is their relationship with this person(s)? Describe how that person typically spends their day.

_____

_____

_____

_____

_____

What causes your loved one stress?

_____

_____

_____

_____

What calms them down when they are stressed or
agitated?

_____

_____

_____

_____

Other information that would help bring joy to your loved
one.

_____

_____

_____

_____

_____

_____

_____

_____

_____

Functional Levels

In addition to the Personal History Form, you also need to look at your loved one's functional level. When planning meaningful activities based on individual interests, you need to also consider your loved one's functional abilities. You need to set them up for success based on what they are able to accomplish. There are several definitions of functional levels. For the purposes of this topic, we will address the following four functioning levels:

Level 1

Your loved one has good social skills. They are able to communicate. They are alert and oriented to person, place and time, and they have a long attention span.

Level 2

Your loved one has less social skills and their verbal skills may be impaired as well. Your loved one may have some behavior symptoms. They may need something to do, and may have an increased energy level, but they have a shorter attention span.

Level 3

Your loved one has less social skills. Their verbal skills are even more impaired than they were at Level 2. They are also easily distracted. Your loved one may have some visual/spatial perception and balance concerns, and they need maximum assistance with their care.

Level 4

Your loved one has a low energy level, nonverbal communication skills, and they rarely initiate contact with others, however, they may respond if given time and cues.

With the personal history and functional level information, you and every caregiver have the greatest opportunity to provide person-appropriate activities for your loved one.

Chapter 5

Communicating and Motivating for Success

Communicating and motivating for success is the Second Pillar for engaging in an activity with your loved one. The key to effective communication is the ability to listen attentively. This requires all caregivers to use communication techniques that provide an open, nonthreatening environment for your loved one. Listening behavior can either enhance and encourage communication or shut down communication altogether. You need to assess your listening style and be able to assess the listening styles of the other caregivers and family members working with your loved one.

Verbal Communication

Communication is an interactive process where information is exchanged. The ability to respond appropriately, or to give feedback, is just as important as having good listening skills.

Verbal Approaches

- Use exact, short, positive phrases. Repeat twice if necessary.

- Speak slowly with words they know.

- Give time for the person to answer.

- Give one instruction at a time.

- Use a warm, gentle tone of voice.

- There is no need to shout, unless the individual also has a hearing impairment.

- If the person is unable to see you because of a visual impairment, be sure to use verbal cues to let them know you are engaged.

- Talk to them like an adult.

Verbal Communication Tips

- Make your presence known when entering a room by saying hello.

- Identify yourself. Do not assume your loved one knows who you are.

- If there are others present, address the person by name so there is no confusion as to whom you are talking to.

- Indicate the end of a conversation and that your loved one knows when you leave.

- Speak directly to your loved one.

- Always answer questions and be specific in your responses.

- When giving directions, make them as simple and clear as possible.

- When speaking with other caregivers about your loved one while they are present, make sure the conversation is respectful of your loved one. They may move or speak slowly, but assume that they hear everything.

Nonverbal Communication

Although it may seem that most communication happens verbally, research has shown that actually most communication occurs nonverbally. Nonverbal communication occurs through an individual's body language. There are five key elements to consider:

Facial Expressions

Be aware of what your facial expressions are conveying to your loved one. Your mood will be mirrored.

Eye Contact

Ensure that you have made eye contact with your loved one and that their attention is focused on you and what you are saying.

Gestures and Touch

Calmly use nonverbal signs such as pointing, waving and other hand gestures in combination with your words.

Tone of Voice

The inflection in your voice helps your loved one relate to the words you are saying.

Body Language

Be aware of the position of your hands and arms when talking to your loved one.

**Note: When communicating with your loved one, be mindful that their body language may not fully tell how they feel or what they are trying to express because of slow movement. Your body language, however, will be read by your loved one.

Nonverbal Communication Tips

- Always approach your loved one from the front before speaking to them.
- Smile and extend your hand as to shake their hand. Use touch where welcomed.
- Be at eye level with the person you are talking to.
- Use nonverbal gestures along with words.

- Give nonverbal praises such as smiles and head nods.

- Be an active listener.

- Make sure that all caregivers give your loved one the opportunity and time to speak.

Being a Detective

As your loved one's dementia progresses, there will be many days that you will not know what kind of day it will be until after it has started. If there is an issue, the starting point in your process is communicating to figure out what they are telling you.

Imagine one morning your loved one wakes up and tells you that someone came into their bedroom in the middle of the night and robbed and raped them. Your first response would be to validate their feelings and to let them know they are now safe. You start the detective work by asking them open-ended questions of who, what, when and where.. Your loved one may not be able to rationalize at the moment, so again, reassure them that they are safe and you are there to protect them.

As you ask questions and have made sure that a stranger did not enter the house in the night, you may realize that it might have been you or another caregiver that went into your loved one's room in the middle of the night to check on them. You might have gone in and you put their clothes away or picked something up off the floor. While you were in the room, you may have noticed they kicked the covers off so you covered them back up. So yes, someone was in your loved one's room and did move their belongings (put clothes away) and yes, someone (you) may have touched them when someone (you) were covering them back up after they had kicked off the blankets.

This is a common accusation and even though every thought deserves for you to be a detective, please remember that your loved one may lose the ability to rationally think through a situation.

Approaches to Successful Communication

<u>Be Calm</u>

Always approach your loved one in a relaxed and calm demeanor. Remember, your mood will be mirrored by your loved one. Smiles are contagious.

<u>Be Flexible</u>

There is no right or wrong way of completing a task. Offer praise and encouragement for the effort your loved one puts into a task. If you see your loved one becoming overwhelmed or frustrated, stop the task and re-approach at another time.

Be Nonresistive

Don't force tasks on your loved one. Adults do not want to be told, "No!" or told what to do. The power of suggestion goes a long way, and you get more with an ounce of sugar than you do a pound of vinegar.

Be Guiding, but Not Controlling

Always use a soft, gentle approach and remember your tone of voice. Your facial expressions must match the words you are saying.

These guidelines are effective and should be followed by you and all family members or other caregivers of your loved one. Let's look at an example of how a common approach by all caregivers can be effective in creating a positive day.

For years, your husband made oatmeal raisin cookies for the family every Sunday afternoon after church. It is one of the happiest memories that your children have of your husband, their father, and their childhood. Everyone was talking, laughing, and enjoying some sweet treats. Your daughter, who now helps you with caregiving duties twice a week, has noticed your husband becoming more withdrawn as he has gotten older and the dementia has progressed. She noticed that the only thing your husband wants to do is sit and watch television. He falls in and out of sleep throughout the day in front of the television, disrupting a normal sleep pattern. Because of that, he constantly wakes himself and you up in the middle of the night causing you to be exhausted during the day. It is a terrible pattern that is wearing you down.

Your daughter remembers the Sunday afternoon cookie making and has tried weekly to get your husband to help make cookies again by asking, "Dad, would you like to make some cookies today?" Your husband always says, "No."

One day, your daughter decides to take a different approach. She knows that your husband loved making the cookies and she knows that your husband loves her son, your grandson, Tommy. Armed with that knowledge, your daughter comes over at noon on her regular caregiving day. After you have left the house to run some errands, she says to your husband, "Dad, I need some help. I am trying to make oatmeal raisin cookies for Tommy and I can't quite get them to come out right. I need someone to make sure I am doing it right, would you help me please?"

Your husband agrees to help your daughter for his grandson's sake. Your daughter tells your husband she has the recipe and that they need to go to the grocery store and then to her house to bake. Your husband becomes nervous and is afraid that it is just a trick to get him out of the house to take him to the nursing home. Your daughter validates his feelings and calmly reassures him that is not the case. She gives him her mobile phone and says that he can call you at any time if he sees that they are not going to the grocery store and then her house to make cookies.

Even though he is a little apprehensive, your husband agrees to go. Once they walk into the grocery store, your daughter begins to pull out the ingredient list and something amazing happens. Your husband looks at her and says, "You do not need that. I know everything we have to get." Moving slowly through the store, they get every ingredient needed to make the cookies.

After leaving the store, they head to your daughter's house and your husband says, "I need to check on your mother." When they arrive at the house, your daughter dials your number and hands the phone to your husband. He tells you that he is helping your daughter make cookies for Tommy and that he just wanted you to know where he was.

After the phone call, your husband and daughter spend a few hours making cookies, talking and laughing. Suddenly your daughter notices your husband becoming very nervous and anxious. He has stopped talking and began pacing in the kitchen. Your daughter, putting on her detective hat, begins asking questions to find out what is wrong. Your husband finally tells her that he needs to call you to let you know that he will be late for dinner. He does not want you to be disappointed with him if you are cooking dinner and it gets cold. The problem is that he cannot remember where you are or how to get in touch with you. Without embarrassing him for not remembering your phone number, your daughter says she can help, picks up the phone and dials your number.

After you assure him that being late or even missing dinner will be okay, your husband has begun talking and laughing with your daughter and her family again. He spends several more hours with them and finally arrives back at your home around 8:30 that evening.

He tells you a little bit about the day, but then says that he is tired and ready for bed. He falls asleep and for the first time in a long time, he sleeps soundly through the night, and so do you.

Planning, patience, effective communication, and the ability to adapt are all easier said than done if you are in the heat of the moment where everything that could happen, does happen.

Armed with the knowledge of your loved one's past and effective communication skills, all caregivers have the opportunity to engage your loved one in a meaningful activity that will improve the quality of your loved one's life and theirs.

Please remember that your loved one did not choose to be here. If they could choose not to have dementia, they would not have it. As the disorder progresses, you may not know what the day is going to hold or even if it will be a good day or a bad day. You must use all of the resources available to you, such as this book, to be ready when it does happen. Accept help when it is offered, and take time to take care of yourself whenever the opportunity arises. As much as it may feel like it at certain times, you are not alone in this fight.

Barriers to Good Communication

There are generally two barriers that negatively affect communication with your loved one. Here are some tips on how to eliminate negative behaviors.

Barriers Created by Caregivers

- Speaking too quickly. Slow down when speaking.
- Use a calm tone of voice and be aware of your hand movements.
- Never be demanding or commanding.
- Never argue with a person with impaired cognition. You will never win the argument.

- Enter their world. Live their truth and validate.
- Do not offer long explanations when answering questions.

Environmental Barriers to Communication

- Noise from air conditioners and home appliances.
- TV on in the same room where you are trying to talk.
- Outside traffic.
- Hearing aid batteries that are whistling.
- Lighting in the room. If the lighting in a room negatively affects your loved one's limited vision, they may be more focused on trying to see rather than on communicating.

Barriers of any type will have a negative effect on communication and could possibly lead to a behavioral issue if your loved one thinks you are yelling at them for no particular reason even though you are trying to be loud enough for them to hear you. Here is an example of something you can try. You have been trying to have a conversation with your loved one. You are making eye contact and standing directly in front of them, but you are still having trouble connecting because the TV is playing in the background and the dogs are barking at the door.

There are three things happening at the same time: your attempt at conversation, the television, and the barking dogs. This can be very overstimulating for your loved one and they do not know where to focus. A good idea would be to address the needs of the dogs and then as you walk into the room smiling, go turn the volume of the television down or turn it off completely while you explain you have a question to ask. You can then sit down at eye level with your loved one before speaking.

Validation of "Living their Truth" as a Tool to Communicating with Someone who has Dementia

For those we care for who have dementia, R.O.S. teaches validation as part of the communication process. Your role when working with your loved one is best expressed by author Jolene Brackey, who preaches that caregivers should take every opportunity to create moments of joy.

Many people struggle with the use of validation. There is a concern that it might appear as if you are lying to your loved one or doing them harm by not keeping them oriented to the truth. In fact, you are not lying to your loved one. You are simply meeting your loved one where they are at this moment and accepting that this is part of the illness.

Let's look at an example of validation. Your loved one is asking for a deceased spouse. Instead of trying to bring them back to reality and causing them to get upset at the news that their loved one is dead, you can keep it simple and say something like, "I have not seen him today" and then give them a reason that makes sense as to where their spouse could be. It might be something like, "You know it is Monday and I bet he is at the printing company working. Let's go have some tea."

Communication and Behavior

Behaviors are a means to communicate when words are no longer effective ...

Behaviors are a means to communicate when words are no longer effective ...

Behaviors are a means to communicate when words are no longer effective!

Caregivers must uncover the meaning behind the behaviors and put a plan into effect to manage those needs. Be a detective.

<u>Aggressive Behaviors</u>

Aggressive behaviors can be defined as hitting, angry outbursts, obscenities, yelling, racial insults, making inappropriate sexual comments and/or biting. Trying to communicate with, or provide care to, a person who is aggressive can be stressful and even frightening for caregivers.

For example, you are engaging in activity with your loved one and everything is going well. Suddenly, out of nowhere your loved one becomes very angry. They begin using profanity while telling you to get out and leave them alone. A good approach would be to validate their feelings and behavior with a simple and calmly spoken comment/question while you are trying to figure out the cause.

"Roger, you seem very angry today. What are you angry about?"

Based on clues presented, you may discover that your loved one feels helpless and is angry about his loss of abilities. This is an opportunity to further validate their feelings and direct the focus to the positives of remaining abilities they do have.

You may have to stop what you were trying to do with your loved one and just focus on their feelings. You may need to give them space and retry the task another time.

Possible Causes for Aggression

- Too much noise or overstimulation
- Cluttered environment
- Uncomfortable room temperatures
- Basic needs not being met: hunger, thirst, needing to use the bathroom, needing comfort
- Pain
- Fear, anxiety or confusion
- Communication barriers
- Fear or anxiety from not recognizing their surroundings

- Caregiver's mood
- Feeling that they are being rushed
- Difficulty seeing activity or materials of activity, which prevents them from participating
- Lack of independence

Interventions to Utilize to Mitigate Aggressive Behaviors

- Validate and support their feelings.
- Reminisce with your loved one about specific details of their past.
- Remain calm and speak in a soft tone.
- Find items that they find comfort in, e.g., a picture of the family.
- Provide consistent caregivers and schedules. Stick to your loved one's routine.
- Engage in recreational activities that match their abilities and interests, as tolerated.

- Break down instructions into one-step increments.

- Identify the triggers of the aggression. Be a detective. There is never a behavior that just occurs.

- Keep an ongoing dialogue between family members and caregivers over any noted changes in patterns or behaviors.

- Help your loved one to slow down and relax.

- Play or listen to music your loved one enjoys for its calming effects.

- Use spiritual support if this is important to your loved one.

Chapter 6

Customary Routines
and Preferences

Customary routines and preferences is the
Third Pillar in an activities program. Activities
can occur all day, every day. The question
should not be, "When should I do activities?"
It is not important to focus on when to do
activities. The focus should be on making
each and every interaction that is a part of
your loved one's daily routine memorable
and enjoyable.

For the purpose of developing a daily plan of
care, we will be discussing two areas: Daily
Customary Routine and Activity Preferences.
The goal is to gain from your loved one's
perspective how important certain aspects
of care/activity are of interest to them as
an individual.

Daily Customary Routine

Your loved one has distinct lifestyle preferences and routines. They should be preserved to the greatest extent possible. All reasonable accommodation should be made to maintain their lifestyle preferences.

Not accommodating your loved one's lifestyle preferences and routine can contribute to a depressed mood and increased behavior symptoms. When a person feels like their control has been removed and that their preferences are not respected as an individual, it can be demoralizing.

Activity Preferences

Activities are a way for individuals to establish meaning in their lives. The need for enjoyable activities does not change based on their age or health needs. The only thing that changes is the level of assistance they may need to engage in those pursuits.

A lack of opportunity to engage in meaningful and enjoyable activities can result in boredom, depression and behavioral disturbances.

Individuals vary in the activities they prefer, reflecting unique personalities, past interest, perceived environmental constraints, religious and cultural background, and changing physical and mental abilities. We as family caregivers have a great opportunity to empower a loved one to see that they possess many great talents and abilities. By modifying or adapting an activity to allow them to engage at an independent level, you are restoring their self-esteem and self-worth.

Chapter 7

Planning and Executing Activities

Planning and executing activities is the Fourth Pillar in engaging a loved one in an activity. With the knowledge of your loved one's history, functional level, effective communication techniques to use, and their daily routine, we now look at planning activities in which they can be successful.

The Lesson Plan

The Lesson Plan template is a guideline for an activity. Each loved one's abilities and responses are different. This will dictate how you modify an activity to meet their individual needs and abilities. The Lesson Plan is an ever-changing document. It is meant to be written on to note any changes needed so the next person working with your loved one can follow your modifications in hopes to recreate a positive experience.

Items in the Lesson Plan

Date

Document the date the program is used.

Program Name

You can rename the program if you or your loved one prefer.

Objective of Activity

Our goal is to provide meaningful activities. People have a need to be productive and they want to engage in something with a purpose. List the objectives of the program.

Materials

The list of suggested materials to use with this program.

Prerequisite Skills

The skills your loved one needs to participate in this program.

Activity Outline

Step-by-step instructions to complete this program.

Evaluation

When you or a family member are conducting an activity with your loved one, documenting results and responses are critical to improve activity programs for your loved one. Items to document:

- Verbal cues, physical assistance or modifications you make to activity.

- Your loved one's response to this program.

- Did your loved one enjoy this activity or not?

- Was the activity successful at distracting or eliminating a negative behavior?

A blank template is included on the next page to give you an example of what a Lesson Plan looks like.

Lesson Plan Blank Example

Date	Program Name

Objective of Activity

Materials

Prerequisite Skills

Activity Outline

Evaluation

Chapter 8

Leisure Activity Categories, Types, Topics and Tips

Activity Categories

Activities are generally broken down into three different categories:

Maintenance Activities

Maintenance activities are traditional activities that help your loved one to maintain physical, cognitive, social, spiritual and emotional health.

Examples include: using manipulative games such as those in the R.O.S. Legacy™ System, craft and art activities, attending church services, working trivia and crossword puzzles like the *How Much Do You Know About* puzzles, taking a walk, and tai chi.

Supportive Activities

Supportive activities are for those that have a lower tolerance for traditional activities. These types of activities provide a comfortable environment while providing stimulation or solace.

Examples include: listening to and singing music, hand massages, relaxation activities such as aromatherapy, meditation and bird-watching.

Empowering Activities

Empowering activities help your loved one attain self-respect by receiving opportunities for self-expression and responsibility.

Examples include: cooking, making memory boxes and folding laundry.

Activity Types

Once you have chosen an activity from a category that will suit your loved one's need, you must choose an activity type that will interest them. There are several types of activities to choose from. Below are some examples:

Art Activities

- Coloring
- Painting
- Dancing

Craft Activities

- Jewelry making
- Knitting
- Scrapbooking

Verbal Activities

- Conversation
- Trivia

Entertainment Activities

- Board games, card games
- Video games
- Crossword puzzles

Listening Activities

- Music
- Storytelling
- Books on tape
- Listening to the radio

Visual Activities

- Watching a movie
- Watching a performance

Writing Activities

- Writing a story or poem
- Writing a letter

Active Activities

- Dancing
- Folding laundry
- Road trips

Activity Topics

Once you know what category of activity you want to engage your loved one from, here are some suggestions for topics the activity can be based on:

Colors

- Colors of their favorite sports team
- Colors of their wedding
- Colors of flowers or cars

Music

- Favorite music
- Music from when they were younger and dating
- Patriotic songs
- Holiday songs
- Favorite artists from the age they think they are, e.g., if they believe they are 25 years old, use popular singers or songs of that era.

Military Service

- War stories
- World events of their time
- Their personal experiences of either military service or what it was like in the States

Holidays

- Specific holidays that coincide with their culture or religion
- Favorite holidays

Cooking

- Home cooking
- Comfort food
- Favorite recipes from their mother/grandmother
- Favorite food associated with events, holidays, family gatherings

Sports

- Professional sports teams they liked
- Their involvement in sports
- Big sporting events from their era

School Days

- Where they went to school
- Favorite school classes or teachers
- Memories of their children's school events

Old Cars

- Their family's first car
- Their first car
- Prices of cars now and then
- Dream cars

Places

- Where they were born
- Where they grew up
- Places they have been
- Vacations they took

**Activity Tips for Individuals
with Mild to Moderate Dementia**

Many loved ones have cognitive deficits that
are significant enough to impact their day as
well as their awareness of their surroundings.

By providing activities that reinforce their past, we increase and improve their social skills which can improve their general interactions with others.

Validating Activities

Validating activities validate the memories and feelings of individuals who are much disoriented. They focus on your loved one's perception of what happened in the past.

Reminiscing Activities

Reminiscing activities are designed to help the client identify the important contributions he or she has made throughout their lifetime. It is an important part of human development to see oneself as a contributing member of society.

Resocializing Activities

Once your loved one can successfully participate in reminiscing and validating activities, it is time to encourage them, through resocializing activities, to build on those social skills and begin to expand their connections to the community in which they live. This can be as simple as with a neighbor, in church, or within their community.

Chapter 9

Activities of Daily Living
Tips and Suggestions

Unlike leisure activities, the Activities of Daily Living covered in this book are necessary activities that are a part of everyday life. The following pages contain tips and suggestions for you to use with your loved one.

Bathing

Bathing can be a relaxing, enjoyable experience or a time of confrontation and anger. Use a calm approach. Your loved one's "usual" routine is very important.

Safety

- Water temperature should range from 110°F to 115°F maximum to prevent burning or skin injury.

- Floor of tub or shower needs skid proofing or a rubber mat.

- Place a nonskid rug on the floor outside the tub to prevent slipping.

- Install grab bars around the tub.

- Do not use bath oils.

NEVER leave your loved one unattended in the bathroom.

Know Your Loved One

- Are they accustomed to a bath or shower?

- Can they get into a bath or shower without assistance?

- Who is your loved one the most comfortable with when needing care? Female/male, a specific caregiver?

NOTE: Sex and age of the caregiver can be a significant issue. For example, a 90-year-old female might be horrified if a 20-year-old male family member came into the bathroom to assist with care. She may fear for her safety or be embarrassed depending on her level of dementia.

Communicating and Motivating

- Don't ask if they want to bathe. Simply say in an easy, friendly voice, "Bath time."

- Use short, simple sentences.

- Look directly at your loved one.

- Be mindful of the little details – preparation and execution.

- Always smile, talk calmly and gently.

- Do not argue, or try to explain "why."

- If your loved one becomes angry or combative about bathing, **STOP** and try another time.

Customary Routines and Preferences

- What time of day does the loved one normally bathe?

- Does your loved one wash their hair or body first?

Planning and Executing

- Consider the process that works for the caregiver and loved one when it is time to bathe.

  For example, your loved one needs assistance undressing and getting into the tub. They always remove their shirt first, followed by their pants, socks and underwear. The tub has a built-in seat that is covered with ceramic tile. Your loved one needs a towel laid on the tile prior to sitting down because the tile is cold against their skin. Once seated, your loved one also likes a towel draped over their shoulders so they feel less exposed with you assisting them while they bathe.

- Have all care items and tools ready prior to starting the bath process.

- Have a shower chair if necessary.

- Have a handheld hose for showering and bathing.

- Have a long-handled sponge or scrubbing brush if they would like to scrub themselves.

- Have sponges with soap inside or a soft soap applicator instead of bar soap. Bar soap can easily slip out of your loved one's hand.

- One step at a time, follow their normal routine. Wash hair first and then wash body, or soak for 10 minutes before washing. When they finish one step, go to the next.

- Remember to STOP and try another time if your loved one becomes angry or combative.

- Have towel and clothing prepared for when the bath is finished.

- Use a terry cloth robe instead of a towel to dry off.

Other Bathroom and Grooming Activities

Brushing Teeth

- Give them step-by-step directions. This may not be as simple as you think. Take a moment and think of all of the steps necessary to brush your teeth, from walking into the bathroom, to finding the toothpaste in the drawer and removing the cap, to rinsing their mouth once they have finished brushing. Depending on your loved one's level of dementia, it might be easier to show them.

- For family members at home, brush your teeth at the same time.

- Use positive reinforcement and compliment your loved one on the good job they are doing.

- Help your loved one to clean their dentures as needed.

Shaving

- Encourage a male to shave.

- Use an electric razor for safety.

- If they need assistance, please provide it.

- Give positive feedback and do not verbally correct.

  For example, if your loved one only managed to shave half of his face, do not criticize and tell them they "did it wrong." Instead, ask if they would like some help.

Makeup

- If your loved one had been accustomed to wearing makeup, there is no reason for this to stop. If she shows interest or desire to wear makeup, encourage her to do so and offer assistance to apply if needed.

Hair

- Try to maintain hairstyle and care as your loved one did.

- Explain each step simply beforehand to reduce any anxiety.

- When washing hair, use nonstinging shampoo.

- Use warm water for washing and rinsing. Tell your loved one before you rinse their hair.

Nails

- Keep nails clean and trimmed. Be gentle while trimming your loved one's nails. Be mindful of how you pull and where you place their fingers and arms.

- If your loved one had a normal/weekly schedule for nail care prior to the onset of dementia or other health issues, please try to maintain that schedule.

- Offer to polish your loved one's nails.

- When polishing, engage your loved one in conversation.

Toileting or Using the Bathroom

- Mark the bathroom door so it can be identified.

- Learn your loved one's individual habits and routines for using the toilet. This may not be something that you know and is part of the changing roles.

- Toilet routinely on rising, before and after meals, and at bedtime at minimum.

- If your loved one is having trouble communicating, please watch for agitation, pulling at their clothes, walking/pacing restlessly. This may be an indication they need to go to the bathroom.

- Assist with clothing as needed and be positive and pleasant while assisting.

- Provide verbal cues/instructions as needed, while being guiding, but not controlling as you do.

Clothing

Know Your Loved One

- Initially, daily clothing choices should remain as they had been and based on your loved one's available wardrobe.

- As their dementia progresses, changes will have to be made. Clothes need to be comfortable and easy to remove, especially to go to bathroom.

Routines and Preferences

- Have a friendly discussion each evening about the next day's schedule and what your loved one may want to wear.

- Remember that as their dementia progresses, changes will have to be made. You may have to limit the choice of clothing and leave only two outfits in their room at a time.

- If your loved one wants to wear the same thing every day, and if you can afford it, buy three or four sets of the same clothing.

- Try to maintain your loved one's preferred dressing routine by laying the clothes out in order of what your loved one prefers to put on first.

Planning and Executing

- Choose clothes that are loose fitting and have elastic waistbands.

- Choose wraparound clothing instead of the pullover type.

- You may consider clothing that opens and closes in the front and not the back for your loved one. This may be helpful in allowing them to dress themselves and maintain some independence.

- Choose clothing with large, flat buttons, zippers or Velcro closures.

- If possible, attach a zipper pull to the end of the zipper to make it easier to zip pants or jackets.

- Choose slip-on shoes and purchase elastic shoelaces that allow shoes to slip on and off without untying the shoelaces.

Dressing

<u>Know Your Loved One</u>

Initially, your loved one may just need verbal cues/instructions on dressing. As their dementia progresses, you will have to take a more active role. Please remember to allow your loved one to dress themselves as long as possible so they can maintain a sense of dignity and independence. You will have to be the judge of when all caregivers need to begin assisting in the dressing process.

Similar to bathing, you need to identify who your loved one is the most comfortable with when needing care. Female/male, a specific caregiver?

Sex and age of the caregiver can be a significant issue.

Communicating and Motivating

- Use short, simple sentences.

- Provide verbal cues/instructions as needed.

- Ask if your loved one would like to go to the toilet before getting dressed.

- If they are confused, give instructions in very short steps, such as, "Now put your arm through the sleeve." It may help to use actions to demonstrate these instructions.

- Give praise as justified to accomplishing each step.

- Always smile, talk calmly and gently.

- Do not argue, or try to explain "why."

- Be guiding, not controlling.

Routines and Preferences

- Does your loved one get dressed first thing in the morning – before breakfast or after breakfast?

- Does your loved one change into pajamas right before bed or after dinner?

- Try to maintain your loved one's preferred routine. For example, they may like to put on all of their underwear before putting on anything else.

Planning and Executing

- Think about privacy – make sure that blinds or curtains are closed and that no one will walk in and disturb your loved one while they are dressing.

- Make sure the room is warm enough to get dressed in.

- Before handing your loved one their clothes, make sure that items are not inside out and that buttons, zips and fasteners are all undone.

- Hand your loved one only one item at a time.

- If needed, let your loved one get dressed while sitting in a chair that has armrests. This will help your loved one keep their balance.

DRESSING NOTE 1: If mistakes are made – for example, something is put on the wrong way – be tactful, or find a way for you both to laugh about it.

DRESSING NOTE 2: It can be useful if your loved one wears several layers of thin clothing rather than one thick layer, as they can then remove a layer if they feel too warm.

DRESSING NOTE 3: Remember that your loved one may no longer be able to tell you if they are too hot or cold, so keep an eye out for signs of discomfort.

Meals

General Information

- Limit distractions. Serve meals in quiet surroundings, away from the television and other activities.

- Your loved one might not be able to tell if something is too hot to eat or drink. Always test the temperature of foods and beverages before serving.

- Keep long-standing personal preferences in mind when preparing food. However, be aware that your loved one may suddenly develop new food preferences or reject foods that were liked in the past.

- Give your loved one plenty of time to eat. It may take an hour or longer to finish a snack or meal.

- Make meals an enjoyable social event so everyone looks forward to the experience.

Eating

Know Your Loved One

- Can your loved one feed themselves?

- Does your loved one have a visual impairment that may affect their ability to see their meal or drink?

  NOTE: Older individuals tend to perceive bright, deep colors as lighter. They are able to see yellow, orange and red more easily than darker colors. Due to change in our eyesight as we age, eating and dining offer additional challenges.

Communicating and Motivating

- Use short, simple sentences.

- Provide verbal cues/instructions as needed.

- Give your loved one your full attention.

- Always smile, talk calmly and gently.

- Do not argue, or try to explain "why."

Routines and Preferences

- No matter what time of day they eat breakfast, lunch and dinner, be consistent everyday.

- Offer snacks throughout the day.

- Do they eat their meals at the kitchen table?

- Limit distractions. Serve meals in quiet surroundings, away from the television and other activities.

- It may take an hour or longer to finish a snack or meal so factor that into the overall schedule of the day.

Planning and Executing

Eating a meal can be a challenge for your loved one with dementia. There are several areas that need to be taken into account such as visual impairment, physical ailment, changes in preferences and dietary restrictions. Here are some simple techniques that can help reduce mealtime problems:

Meal Preparation for Mild Dementia

- If your loved one wants to assist in making a meal:

  o Make sure your cabinets are organized with each item labeled with large easy-to-see labels.

  o Use simple step-by-step written or verbal instructions.

  o You or another caregiver should perform tasks using sharp objects such as knives, or operation of the stove or oven.

  o When using a stove top, use the back burners and turn the pot handles inward toward the back of the stove to avoid any potential grabbing of the pots or pans.

- If you are not there to supervise because you have to go to work:

  o Avoid planning meals that require use of the stove. Your loved one may not remember to turn off the stove and may not be able to distinguish between a pot that is hot or cold.

- o Lay out the ingredients of a meal on the counter or in the refrigerator in labeled containers in the order that your loved one will use them (similar to laying out their clothes at night).

- o Transfer bulk items, including milk, from a larger container to a smaller container that is easier to lift and pour.

Meal Preparation for Higher Level Dementia

- Try to have all meals eaten at a kitchen or dining table, or a chair with a serving tray. Avoid meals in bed, if possible. Let the bed be for sleeping.

Appropriate Lighting and Eyesight

- Reduce glare by having your loved one sit with the sunlight behind them when eating.

- Use lighting which illuminates the entire dining space and makes objects visible, as well as reducing shadows or reflections.

- Adjust lighting above the table to help see as much detail as possible.

- Remember that older individuals tend to perceive bright, deep colors as lighter. They are able to see yellow, orange and red more easily than darker colors.

Setting the Table and Serving

- Set each place setting in the same way for every meal. Set it the way your loved one used to, and offer them the opportunity to assist in setting the table.

- Decide how to set the rest of the table – main dish, side dishes, seasonings and condiments. Do it the same way each day.

- When pouring a light-colored drink, such as milk, use a dark glass.

- When pouring a dark-colored drink, such as cola, use a white glass.

- Avoid clear glasses. They can disappear from view.

- Use white dishes when eating dark-colored food and use dark dishes when eating light-colored food.

- To make dishes easier to find on the table, use a tablecloth or placemats that are the opposite color of the dishes.

- Fiesta ware colors (yellow/tangerine) contrast with most foods so they can be easily seen and will enhance visual perception.

- There should be a clear visual distinction between the table, the dishes and the food.

- Use solid colors with no distracting patterns.

Chapter 10

Review

Activities can improve the quality of life of both you and your loved one. There are many benefits to an activity program for your loved one and you have the opportunity to enjoy them all.

Now that we have gone through the items necessary to put together a successful activity program, let us review the Four Pillars of a successful program one last time.

1st Pillar of Activities:
Know Your Loved One – Information Gathering and Assessment

Have a Personal History Form completed. Know them – who they are, who they were, and what their functional abilities are today. Make sure all caregivers know this as well.

<u>2nd Pillar of Activities:</u>
Communicating and Motivating for Success

Communication is key. Each caregiver must know how to effectively communicate with your loved one and be consistent with techniques.

<u>3rd Pillar of Activities:</u>
Customary Routines and Preferences

As best as possible, maintain a routine and daily plan based on your loved one's needs and preferences.

<u>4th Pillar of Activities:</u>
Planning and Executing Activities

Based on all of the information you have gathered about your loved one, you have the opportunity to offer engaging activities that are appropriate and meet your loved one's personal preferences.

About the Authors

Scott Silknitter

Scott Silknitter is the founder of R.O.S. Therapy Systems.
He designed and created the R.O.S. Play Therapy™ System,
the *How Much Do You Know About* Series of themed
activity books and the R.O.S. *BIG Book*. Starting with
a simple backyard project to help Mom and Dad,
Mr. Silknitter has dedicated his life to improving the quality
of life for all seniors through meaningful education,
entertainment and activities.

Robert D. Brennan, RN, NHA, MS, CDP

Robert Brennan is a Registered Nurse and Nursing Home
Administrator with over 35 years of experience in long-
term care. He is a Certified Dementia Practitioner and is
Credentialed in Montessori-Based Dementia Programming
(MBDP) providing general and Train the Trainer programs.
Robert was responsible for the development of an Assisted
Living Federation of America (ALFA) "Best of the Best"
award-winning program for care of individuals with
dementia using MBDP. He currently provides education on
dementia and long-term regulatory topics.

Dawn Worsley, ADC/MC/EDU, CDP

Dawn Worsley is a Certified Activity Director with a specialization in Education and Memory Care, a Certified Eden Alternative Associate, and a Certified Dementia Practitioner. With over 20 years of experience, Ms. Worsley is an authorized certification instructor with the National Certification Council of Dementia Practitioners and a Modular Education Program for Activity Professionals course instructor.

References

1. *The Handbook of Theories on Aging* (Bengtson et al., 2009)
2. *Activity Keeps Me Going, Volume 1* (Peckham et al., 2011)
3. *Essentials for the Activity Professional in Long-Term Care* (Lanza, 1997)
4. *Abnormal Psychology*, Butcher
5. www.dhspecialservices.com
6. National Certification Council for Dementia Practitioners www.NCCDP.org
7. "Managing Difficult Dementia Behaviors: An A-B-C Approach" By Carrie Steckl
8. Iowa Geriatric Education Center website, Marianne Smith, PhD, ARNP, BC Assistant Professor University of Iowa College of Nursing
9. *Excerpts taken from "Behavior...Whose Problem is it?" Hommel, 2012
10. *Merriam-Webster's Dictionary*
11. "The Latent Kin Matrix" (Riley, 1983)
12. *Care Planning Cookbook* (Nolta et al.2007)
13. "Long-Term Care" (Blasko et al. 2011)
14. "Success Oriented Programs for the Dementia Client" (Worsley et al 2005)
15. Heerema, Esther. "Eight Reasons Why Meaningful Activities Are Important for People with Dementia." www.about.com
16. *Activities 101 for the Family Caregiver* (Appler-Worsley, Bradshaw, Silknitter)
17. American Foundation for the Blind
18. www.aging.com
19. www.WebMD.com
20. www.caregiver.org

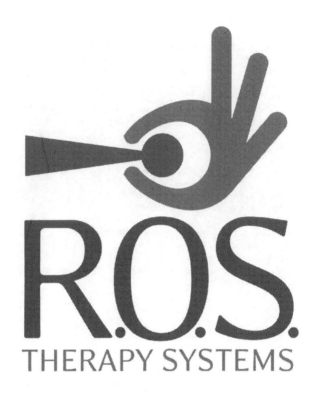

For additional assistance, please contact us at:
www.ROSTherapySystems.com
888-352-9788

Made in the USA
Middletown, DE
20 October 2015